Women Of Iron

Empowerment Through Strength Training!

RON KNESS

Contents

Disclaimer

This publication is for informational purposes only and is not intended as medical advice. Medical advice should always be obtained from a qualified medical professional for any health conditions or symptoms associated with them.

Every possible effort has been made in preparing and researching this material. We make no warranties with respect to the accuracy, applicability of its contents or any omissions.

See your healthcare professional before starting any diet or exercise program!

Introduction

Unfortunately, some women may consider muscle building or strength training to be an activity exclusively meant for men, however nothing can be further from the truth. It's a sad fact that the National Center for Health Statistics reports only 21% of ladies hit the iron section of the gym and strength train two or more times a week.

Women who perform weight training enjoy better health and often improve the look of their body. One of its best benefits is the more lean muscle mass your body has, the more fat it burns naturally, even when the body is at rest because it is muscle that burns fat!

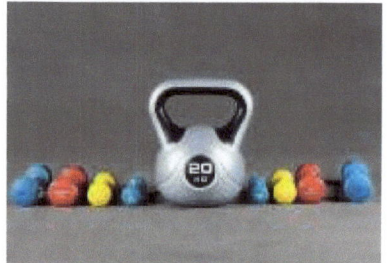

Moreover, weight training improves aging, and allows you to remain strong and both mentally and physically competent as the consequences of time come knocking.

Besides, ladies, nothing looks more cool or hot than slapping on the weight gloves and pumping iron, it makes you feel strong, capable, and empowered! To the point that you feel you can do anything!

It is important to note that weight training comes in many levels, and the lifting done for general health is completely different from the type that women bodybuilders perform.

In fact, it would take quite a bit of very deliberate effort and specific technique to get as big as those women who choose to become bodybuilders do.

The type of weight training that targets general health is for *any* woman who wants to build lean muscle mass, and reap the numerous health benefits that it offers at any age.

Many women shy away from strength training because they think they will "bulk up" like men do. That is completely false, because women just do not have the necessary amount of testosterone it takes to build large muscles. The women that do bulk up normally take a "T" supplement. What you will get are tone and defined muscles, plus you'll naturally burn more calories because of the additional toning.

Weight Training and Its Goals

Weight training is any strength training exercises where weights are used for resistance – dumbbells, barbells and kettlebells all qualify. Weight training stresses or shocks muscles, and this causes them to grow and get stronger by adapting to the environment created during lifting. They don't like the stress put on them, so they grow (slightly) to relieve the stress.

The truth is muscle is either growing, shrinking or staying the same. Weight training strengthens muscles much in the same way that running, cycling, or any cardio strengthens the heart. When you lift weights, you not only build lean muscle mass, you 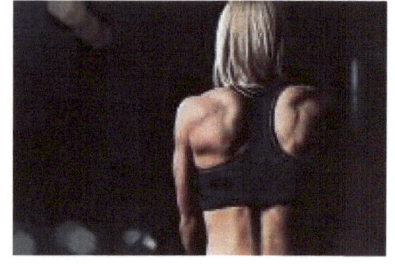 improve your physical and mental strength as well. All of a sudden, daily chores, such as doing laundry, carrying in groceries and vacuuming become easier with your newfound strength.

Weight training uses resistance against the force of gravity to create an opposition in force generated by muscle, through either concentric or eccentric contraction.

Besides, the types of weights already mentioned, muscle building can be accomplished with "weight machines" found at the gym or home gyms that simulate real weight, resistance bands and even by using your own body for resistance, such as the case in bodyweight exercise moves.

Weight Training Verses Other Types of Training

There are many types of different exercise, including:

- Endurance/aerobic training

- Cardio, such as walking, jogging, elliptical or cycling

- Anaerobic training, such as HIIT and Tabata

- Flexibility exercises, such as yoga and pilates

- Balance training

- Strength training - Strength training is an inclusive term used to describe any exercise move that's goal is to increase physical strength. Weight training is one such example that uses weight for resistance. Resistance bands is another example, but it does not use weight.

While weight training has become synonymous with strength training, it is actually a more specific type of exercise within the inclusive category that offers many real and significant benefits for women of all ages.

13 Benefits of Weight Training for Women

There are numerous health benefits in gaining lean muscle mass besides looking and feeling great.

Long Term Bone Health

Women are especially vulnerable to bone deterioration later in life, such as osteoporosis. There may be ways to prevent or lessen bone health problems altogether, one of which is the principle of biomechanics called Wolff's Law.

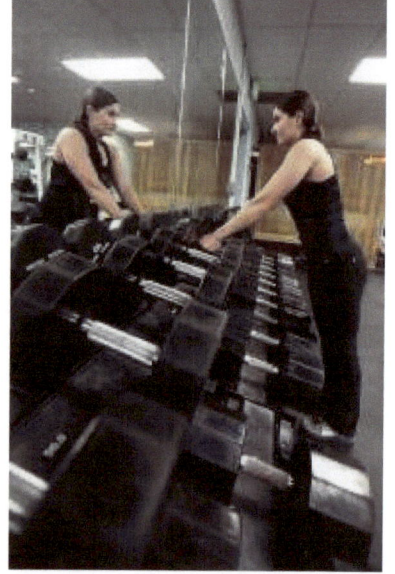

Wolff's Law states that applying a bending force, such as a muscle contraction of physical load on a bone stimulates the bone remodeling process causing bone to grow thicker and stronger over time to adapt to the stress.

Stop and consider this for a moment. This is literally the exact opposite of a bone wasting condition that occurs naturally as women age.

Therefore, weight lifting is beneficial for any woman wanting to strengthen the bones and especially for those who have a family history of osteoporosis.

Calorie Burning

Most women choose slow steady state cardio as their default calorie burning activity. However, cardio is quickly becoming old news in the fat burning quest and is being replaced by high intensity interval activity (HIIT) and weightlifting, both of which are anabolic and licit a response called EPOC (excess post-exercise oxygen consumption).

EPOC occurs as result of the high anaerobic state of intense exercise. Basically, oxygen is squeezed out of the muscle and it takes 24-36 hours to replenish that lost O_2. During that time period, resting metabolic rate is drastically increased, meaning you are burning more calories than normal.

This results in a significant increase in Resting Metabolic Rate many hours after intense exercise that is just too significant to ignore. This is known as "afterburn".

Increase In Lean Body Mass

Celebrity trainer Jillian Michaels has a really good definition of lean body mass: "Women should have a body fat of 20 to 21%, meaning that the rest of their body composition will be lean tissue - organs, muscle, bone and water." In this definition, lean body mass is not just the absence of fat, in fact, a healthy body will have about 20% body fat and lean muscle mass.

Lean body means having an abundance of lean tissue. Without all these things in good proportion, the body simply doesn't function correctly. Weight lifting supports lean body mass, by lowering body fat levels and increasing muscle mass.

Reduced Cancer Risk

The *Idea Fitness Journal* (2015) notes women with a higher lean body mass are 41% less likely to develop cancer than those with higher body fat percentages; this study was focused on obese women who typically have higher body fat percentage.

Knowing that lowering your body fat and increasing your

lean body mass can reduce your cancer risk by 41% should be enough for anyone to see the benefits of having a lean body. Cancer is very prevalent in our society, and 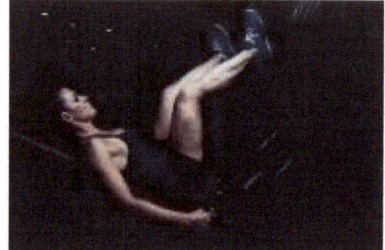 anything you can do to reduce that risk is worth the effort.

Lower Mortality

Today half the advertisements we see on TV here are focused on living a longer healthier life. You don't have to purchase any products to find the fountain of youth. The Department of Internal Medicine at Seoul National University conducted a study that showed higher Lean Mass Index (LMI) and not lower Body Mass Index (BMI) was key in survival in elderly populations. The higher LMI a person has, the more likely they were to survive to greater ages. BMI, a ratio of weight to height, has been used to calculate mortality risks since its invention.

New studies are showing mortality risks are less about BMI ratio, but better assessed through the amount of lean body mass a person holds.

This new information has correlated with what the fitness industry has been saying for a long time: BMI is biased against the person who has volume of muscle mass because muscle weighs more than fat, a person with a high LMI is going to present a high BMI and the two are contradictory when examining survival rates. Lean body mass is calculated by using a formula that takes body weight minus body fat. The three popular formulas are the Boer, James and Hume. Goggle them to see the calculations of each.

Increased Metabolism

A joint study with University of Alabama and Queensland University of Technology showed that lean body mass was the key indicator in resting metabolic rate (the rate at which you burn calories when at rest) differences between people of the same age and weight.

While the study focused on racial differences in lean body mass to illustrate the point, the primary factors in the racial differences were an increase in lean body mass associated with skeletal long bone differences. The increase in bone and muscle mass led to an increased LMI. This was why there were higher resting metabolic rates.

Muscle Burns Fat! The more muscle mass you have on your body, the more fat you burn even when at rest. By the way, this also includes belly fat, which is visceral fat, a most dangerous type of fat linked to risks of premature death in a direct correlation with waist size.

Confidence

There are very few things in life that mimic the feeling of absolutely crushing a new personal record on weight lift. The ability to quantify and see increases in your physical strength will definitely transfer over into your confidence and overall positive psychological state.

Consider that once you have achieved some incredible milestone, like a 200lb. deadlift, how on earth could anything in real life "weigh you down?"

Prevent Boredom

Cardio is boring - really it is. The only variety is changing machines or methods. Weight lifting allows you unlimited variations, and numerous exercise options, so you never get bored and anything you can do to keep your training fresh will ensure a much higher level of adherence for the long term. Because you should not work the same muscle group two days in a row, it actually forces you to do different routines, which not only work different muscles, but involve different moves, thus preventing boredom.

When you weight train, you will gain strength in your muscles, even if those muscles don't increase in size. Weight training not lonely balances the physique, but improves and increases blood circulation. Helps fight and eliminate cellulite.

It's Just Plain Cool!

If the above is not enough to convince you, this might: Weight lifting is just plain cool and you will look very hot sweating over iron next to the muscle dudes at the gym, all day, and every day!

Unless your doctor advises you otherwise, it is never too late to build muscle mass.

Experts advise that the human body begins to lose 1% of lean muscle mass per year after age 40, so maintaining strength and muscle mass becomes a much more critical consideration as you age to improve your everyday performance, maintain a healthy weight, and for bone health, and general strength.

Additionally, it's scary to imagine that when you hit your 40s, 50s and beyond, your metabolism also begins to slow naturally, and many find themselves suddenly packing on the pounds even when they have not changed their regular diet in any way. The only other way to not gain weight is to reduce your caloric consumption at the same rate as your metabolism slows down … unless you strength train!

Consider the fact that overlooking that weight room means you miss out on a key fat burning advantage.

Just **two weight lifting sessions per week can actually reduce your overall body fat by around 3% in just ten weeks**' time, even if you do not change your diet in anyway and help you to achieve or maintain a lean and toned body.

So, please go ahead and hit those weights regardless of your age, it's never too late to start and you won't regret it!

Weight Training Workouts

Here are some examples of different workouts and exercises you can use to build strength and muscle, and possibly incorporate into your weight training routine.

Free Weights And Weight Machines

Free weights or dumbbells are used to perform various weight lifting exercise and they come in various weight options, as low as 2 pounds to over 35 pounds each.

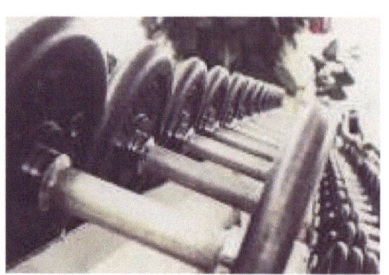

In the free weights category, there are also barbells, which are long metal bars to which disks of varying weights are attached at each end.

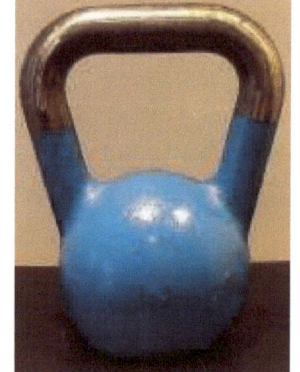

Kettlebells are another type of free weight that have a unique handle and come in various sizes.

There are also weight machines at the gym that work all the parts of the body.

Examples Of Weight Training Exercises

This list is not inclusive, and there are many other moves you can do when weight training.

Dumbbell Bench Press

These are great for you to work both your chest and arms. They are done by laying on your back on a bench with feet placed on the ground. With a dumbbell size you can easily handle in each hand, place your arms near your chest then extend them straight up into the air.

Dumbbell Rows

This popular exercise is just like rowing a boat with oars as the name implies. It will work your arms, chest and back muscles. Start by spreading your feet shoulder width apart. Hold the dumbbells near your waist in front of you with your fingers pointing down. While keeping your fingers pointing down still, bring the dumbbells up to your chest and repeat for several reps.

Dumbbell Pullover

This exercise requires only a single dumbbell. Lay on the bench again with your back resting on it and your feet flat on the ground on either side of the bench (or you can also use a large exercise ball to lay on). Start with your hands straight up in the air holding the dumbbell. Then slowly lower it in one fluid motion so the dumbbell goes down behind your head. This exercise will work your arms very well.

Reverse Laterals

This exercise is somewhat like dancing with dumbbells. While holding the dumbbells in your hand at your sides, step laterally alternating legs and do a reverse lunge as you do it. At the same time alternate raising the opposite side arm from the leg, you are reverse lunging with at that time.

This will work several parts of your body very nicely.

Adductor Squats

This is another weight training exercise that uses only a single dumbbell. You grab the dumbbell and place it in front of you waist high with your feet shoulder width apart. Bend your knees and squat while keeping your back straight and arms locked. It will work your legs and buttocks.

CrossFit™

CrossFit™ training is exactly what the name implies. You will use a broad spectrum of exercises to accomplish your fitness goals and it specifically targets functional fitness, which means that the exercises are designed to mimic everyday life activities, which is the functional part to make you stronger and able to better perform when reaching, bending, and even tying your shoes. Many CrossFit™ training exercises use weights, bodyweight, kettlebells, and even giant tires to build strength and teach the muscles to work together.

There are many CrossFit™ gyms around the country, and it is important to learn the moves in a proper way with instruction and guidance of a qualified CrossFit™ trainer.

CrossFit™ Exercise Examples

Back Squats

This is a great leg and back workout. You start out in a squatting position with the barbell resting on the back of your neck. Raise yourself up using just your legs and not moving your arms at all.

Overhead Presses

This is an exercise that will work your arms, shoulders, and back. You start out in a standing position with your feet shoulder width apart. At the same time, you will rest the barbell on your chest. Using just your arms, you will then lift the barbell above your head until your arms are fully extended.

Deadlifts

These work several muscle groups in your body. Start out with a barbell on the floor in front of you. Squat down and grab the barbell with your fingers facing the floor. Force yourself up with your legs while keeping your back straight. Stop when the weight gets to your hips.

Power Clean

This exercise works the entire body and is an elemental CrossFit™ move. You will start in a squat position with a barbell in your hands on the floor in front of you. You will then proceed to a standing position with the barbell at your waist. Once there you will then raise the barbell above your head until your arms are fully extended.

Barbell Thruster

This is an intense CrossFit™ exercise. You start in a squatting position with a barbell resting on your chest and shoulders. All in one motion spring up with your legs and raise the barbell up at the same time until your arms are fully extended over your head once you stand up straight. This exercise will again work several different muscle groups.

Bodyweight Exercises

Both men and women use bodyweight training as a successful part of any fitness routine. Bodyweight training usually carries less risk of injury with it than regular weight training, but the exercises must still be done correctly to benefit from them.

Examples Of Bodyweight Exercises

Inclined Pushups

These tend to be a little bit easier on the body than regular pushups. They are done by placing your hands on an elevated object such as a bench with your toes still touching the floor. Next, push yourself up using just your arms. Proper form when you are doing an inclined pushup includes making sure your palms are placed directly below your armpits. Declined push-ups puts more pressure on your arms by shifting your weight forward. Instead of having your arms elevated, you have your feet instead. This exercise works the shoulders, arms, and chest.

Bench Dips

This is a good exercise that will work the shoulders and triceps. Again, you will need a bench or something similar to rest your hands on. You will put both hands behind you about shoulder-width apart with your fingers facing toward you. Lower your body up and down using your arms only.

Pull-ups

This traditional exercise can really benefit your shoulders and biceps. You will need a bar that is placed higher than you are tall. Put your hands on the bar a little less than shoulder length apart with your fingers facing toward you. Let your body hang and pull yourself up using only your arms. As a variation, have your fingers pointing away from you. These are called chin-ups. Pull-ups and chin-ups are advanced training moves that takes quite a bit of upper body strength.

Squats

The squat is one of the most beneficial exercise moves known to man. Lower body training does not have to be as complicated as people make it out to be. Squats will give your glute's and legs an excellent workout. They also support joint health, and bone strength.

These are done by standing with your legs hip-width apart and extending your arms straight out in front of you for balance. Bend at the knees and lower your body until your upper thighs are parallel to the floor.

Get back to the starting position by pushing yourself back up using your quads. To increase the difficulty, squats can be done holding dumbbells for increased resistance. For heavier dumbbells, keep your arms down.

Knee Tucks

These are very similar to crunches and sit-ups, but easier on your body. They are great for working your abs and other muscles in your midsection.

You start by lying on your back and bringing your knees up to your chest then alternate between extending your legs straight out and then back to your chest again.

Considerations for Building Muscle

Here are your key considerations when you want to build strength and transform your body.

Scale Weight Versus Body Fat

Muscle weighs more than fat. This is the reason that you hear muscle builders talk about putting on weight; they are referring to muscle mass.

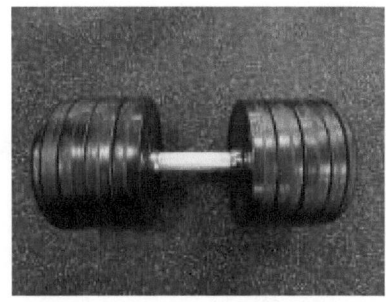

In fact, most weight trainers rarely consider their scale weight, but rather measure body fat using a fat caliper as that is much more representative of the true picture of a muscular body and lean body mass than a scale.

A woman may be 10 to 15 pounds overweight by scale standards, but if she only has 20% body fat, and lean muscle mass, she is 100% fit.

Designing Your Workout

There are many ways to design an ideal workout that ranges from focusing on one or two body parts per day to a schedule where each body part is only trained two times per week.

Beginners are best served with a full body program that takes place 3 days per week, or possibly a 2-day split program done two times per week.

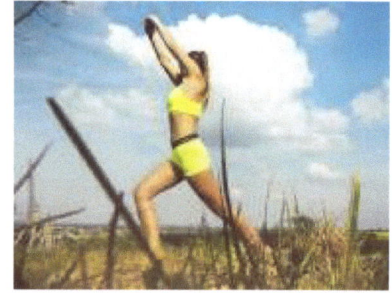

As you advance, you can tweak the design of your workout to suit your individual goals and needs and to possibly concentrate on specific muscle groups that you may want to target.

For example, Mondays for triceps and chest, Wednesdays for the legs and Sundays for the back and biceps. An important point is to not work the same muscle groups two consecutive days in a row. The muscles need at least a day of rest to repair and recover.

When choosing this type of schedule, keep in mind that many lifts are compound, where multiple muscle groups are worked at the same time, so you will want to avoid overlap to allow those muscle groups to get sufficient recovery time between workouts.

Get A Personal Trainer

A certified personal trainer can assist you in creating a workout plan just for you, and teach you how and what to lift to stay safe and boost your results.

All gyms offer personal training and many provide free sessions with membership.

Various Stages of Muscle Building

Hypertrophy

Hypertrophy is the stage in weight lifting where the most muscle growth occurs. Typically, a Hypertrophy Program will last about 4 to 6 weeks, while this is the state where the most muscle growth occurs, and this may seem scary, it is essential to build a solid foundation and to prime the stabilizer and major muscle groups.

Strength

Strength is the second stage in training where there is little to no change in the actual size of muscle. Progress is monitored by the amount of weight being lifted.

Typically, workouts are varied every 2 to 4 weeks to ensure that both major and small muscle groups are being worked.

Endurance

An *Endurance Training* stage is used in fat loss (cutting) programs and involves building lean muscle with high reps and lower rest times between sets.

Power Training

The *Power Training* stage focuses on building explosive strength using lower rep ranges and longer rest periods between sets.

Alternating between Endurance and Power Training stages will keep the body guessing and shock it into a new challenge.

How Much Weight?

Make sure you use appropriate weight as a beginner to avoid injury. You can increase the weight as you get stronger. Typically, if you can easily do 10 reps with a weight, it is too light. If the last rep is difficult to do, you are lifting about the right amount of weight.

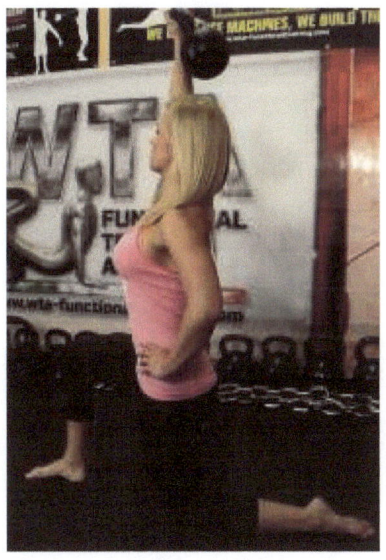

As a general rule of weight training, you do not want to succeed with every set. Lifting should be a struggle, if it too easy, it means the weight is not heavy enough, giving the body the message that it can handle it, and that it does not need to grow more muscle mass and improve.

You don't want to ask your body to deliver, you want to force it to adapt.

Adaptation means the body needs to grow stronger and build more muscle mass to survive and get rid of the stress.

Take the time to focus on and putting sufficient energy into your lifting routine. The weight should be heavy enough to cause micro tears in the muscle tissue that will rebuild stronger and bigger during times of rest, a process referred to a hypertrophy.

Safety should also be a top concern, so it is important to use the correct weight for your fitness level and to perform the exercises in a safe and careful manner to avoid injury, a personal trainer can be of great help in this regard.

Reps & Sets

Rep (repetition) → one complete motion of an exercise

Set → a group of consecutive repetitions

For building muscle mass, an 8-12 rep range, not including warm-ups with 2 to 5 sets per specific exercise will yield good results. As you advance, you will be able to perform more sets.

Shock The Muscle

The body is a miracle of adaptation, no matter what you throw at it, its only goal is to do whatever it needs to survive and succeed, so in order for training to be effective on a continuous basis, you have to challenge your body and shock the muscle by periodically changing your routine.

Rule of thumb: If it's too easy, it's time to upgrade:

- Use fewer sets

- Add weight

- Add new exercises

- Alternate between power and endurance lifting

- Turn to more advanced principles including, compound sets, or drop sets that will quickly shock your body and get it back into a growth stage to further propel your results

Rest break time between sets will depend greatly on the type of lifting you are doing and its goals.

Rest and Recovery Between Workouts

Muscle grows during recovery and rest periods and not actually during lifting, which is why rest periods are critical in effective weight training.

Insufficient recovery time results in further muscle breakdown with each workout that causes a decrease in both their size and strength.

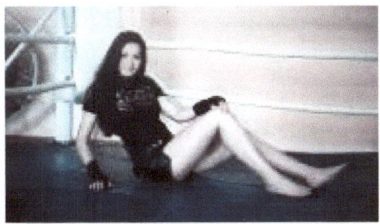

The main consideration is to fine-tune a balance between workouts that progressively overloads the muscles and rest periods that allow them to heal.

It is key to remember that it is during recovery that muscle grows.

Recovery: The Time Factor

Consider your general lifestyle when planning your workouts. If you have a desk job, you will be sedentary more of the time so you will recover faster. But if you have a physically taxing job, you will recover slower and will need more rest time between training sessions.

Proper Form

One of the most important, if not the most important consideration in weight training, is to learn and maintain proper form at all times with any lifting moves you do.

This is critical in avoiding injury and to get the best possible results in muscle growth.

2 Approaches To Building Muscle Mass

There are two major approaches to gaining muscle mass:

- A moderate approach where you bulk much slower, while maintaining or even losing body fat.

- Cutting (fat loss) phase first followed by mass bulking phase where the focus is entirely on building muscle with which comes the inevitable result of gaining some fat mass along the way.

"Bulking" (muscle growth) means a caloric surplus, while "cutting" (losing body fat) means a caloric deficit.

In short, the physiological properties that are responsible for increasing muscle size and strength (anabolism) and the mechanisms responsible for fat loss (catabolism) are not wide-open eight lane highways; they are more like a one-way street.

You can't be in a state of catabolism and anabolism at the same time, it's either one or the other.

Obviously the two are very different, as someone who is overweight or obese will want to strike a balance between losing body fat and gaining some lean muscle, while the woman with a low body fat level may want to focus much more on muscle growth.

The main difference between both methods is the cardio and nutrition elements.

Separating Cardio And Weight Training

An important fact to keep in mind is that weight training does

not, nor should it, replace other workouts, like cardio or HIIIT (high intensity interval training).

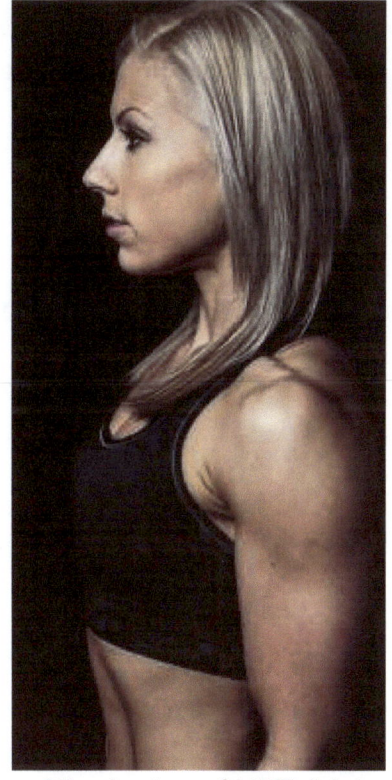

Remember, that each has its own specific benefits and uses. While cardio strengthens the heart and helps to maintain a healthy weight, weight training builds strength and lean muscle mass.

However, cardio can slow down the bulking (muscle building) process, and greatly depends on the intensity and duration of the cardio being performed.

Excessive cardio equals more than 45 minutes of steady cardio or 30 minutes of HIIT (high intensity interval training).

After these amounts of time the body becomes catabolic, which means it begins to eat muscle for fuel instead of dietary intake or even worse the body's fat stores.

This is not only counterproductive to muscle building, but it also sabotages weight loss or even weight maintenance efforts as reducing lean muscle mass also slows metabolism, which may increase body fat levels.

You can also become catabolic when you don't eat enough calories, something women often fall victim to when following disastrous fad diets that are based on starvation, which are never healthy and set you up for failure, as they can never be maintained for the long term.

Another important consideration is never do cardio after a muscle-building workout when your body is drained, a time when you need to replenish energy stores with some type of protein so the muscles can begin to recover and grow, instead of destroying them further.

High Intensity Interval Training

HIIT is anabolic training; cardio is endurance training. HIIT is a better option than traditional slow and steady cardio where you expend energy at a continuous level for a set amount of time (endurance).

HIIT is an anabolic workout that involves intervals of strenuous activity followed by short periods of slower activity or rest. Anabolism is the opposite of breaking down, it is building up versus the catabolic state, which is its complete opposite and requires no energy to occur.

And guess what? Muscle building is also an anabolic activity.

Doing 20-minute HIIT sessions one to three times per week is a better option and of course, the times per week depend on the goals of fitness, fat loss versus gaining muscle mass.

The shorter but intense HIIT workout will not give the body mixed messages as to the muscle fibers you are hoping to train; fast twitch fibers called upon during weight training versus slow twitch fibers targeted during long endurance cardio sessions.

This is one of the reasons that serious runners are usually not very muscular, but have a more stringy look to their bodies.

When building muscle you always want to target the fast twitch muscle fibers so you want to keep any cardio sessions short, but intense, and the perfect solution is HIIT at around 20 minutes per session.

With HIIT being so intense, it also offers the added benefit of creating an anabolic environment, which is similar to weight training encouraging further muscle growth instead of breaking it down as seen during endurance training.

High intensity training does not burn fat during the workout, but revs the body's metabolism all day every day, just like weight lifting does.

The HIIT Equation

HIIT will not break down muscle mass; it is more effective for fat burning as it continues to burn fat for 24 hours or more after a workout even when the body is at rest.

This makes HIIT a better choice over cardio as it reduces the chances of gaining body fat during the calorie surplus bulking phase.

During the bulking phase, HIIT will also deliver key nutrients to growing muscles through the intense increase in blood flow throughout the body, which aids in recovery and growth of muscles mass

HIIT also supports heart health and makes it strong so you don't have to worry about this angle when you switch from cardio to HIIT.

Bottom Line

Consider your cardio choices carefully and take the time to evaluate your total training program to create workout sessions that compliment it.

Diet and Calorie Considerations

Muscles need food to grow, period. Remember that bulking (muscle growth) means a caloric surplus, while cutting (losing body fat) means a caloric deficit.

When your goal is to grow muscles, you will need precious calories, even more calories than you need to maintain daily activities.

This is another reason to choose short HIIT sessions where you will not be burning massive amounts of energy and that which you do burn can easily be replaced in your diet.

Feeding Muscle: Pre and Post Workout

Muscles need energy to grow and building muscle is a very energy consuming process that requires the right kind of building blocks to see results. The post and pre-workout food is most important.

Whey Protein

Whey protein is the translucent liquid visible when the casein protein (curd), is separated in the process of making cheese. Exercise physiologist Fabio Comana of the National Association of Sports Medicine, and many fitness experts report that whey protein has the most amino acids and is easy to digest.

Whey protein supplements are available in their purest form, *whey protein isolate*, which is created by a filtration process that removes the lactose and ash from the original whey protein.

The main differences between the isolate and non-isolate form of whey protein is the actual fat, lactose, and protein content.

Whey protein powder contains:

- 11 to 14.5% protein

- 63 to 75% lactose

- 1 to 1.5% milk fat

Whey protein isolate contains:

- More than 90% protein

- 0.5% of lactose and milk fat

Consuming about 6 grams of essential amino acids with 35 grams of carbohydrates right before exercise will optimize muscle protein synthesis by as much as 200% above resting level.

Whey protein has lactose, a carbohydrate glucose (milk sugar) that maybe beneficial in providing lasting and quick access energy for the muscles so you can perform during intense workouts.

Additionally, according to the article, "**Protein Intake: Effect of Timing**" by Dr. Jay R. Hoffman, research has shown that a carbohydrate load before workouts can increase the amount of amino acids your muscles are able to absorb.

However, many prefer the whey isolate due it to its very high protein concentration. You can also add carbs to a whey protein isolate shake by mixing it with milk or having it with a piece of fruit.

Pre And Post Lifting Nutrition Recommendations

Have a shake with 30 grams of protein and some type of quick-acting carb, like glucose from dairy 30 minutes before a lifting workout to put the body into an anabolic state.

The rest of the above shake should be drank within 30 minutes after the lifting is over. About 35 minutes after that shake, have another small snack with a healthy carb and another ½ portion of the protein shake.

One hour after the last snack, it is time for a complex carb, such as a 1/4 cup of steel cut oatmeal and a protein, like a 1/2 cup of Greek yogurt or cottage cheese.

The above are just examples, as you can have a 3-ounce chicken breast to cover the protein, just as long as you have similar small meals after the workout that will reverse the breakdown of muscle mass, but are still small enough to prevent the food from being stored as fat inside the body.

The main point is that you need protein to support muscle growth.

General Nutrition Is Key

It is amazing how some people can spend hours in the gym, training and sweating and then they eat like total idiots. No matter how good your training, if your diet is not healthy you will not see the results you are looking for. You can't out-exercise a bad diet!

Protein

Protein is the first priority when building muscle because it is the building blocks of muscle mass. Eat a little protein with each meal. Typically 1 1/2 grams of protein per pound of bodyweight is recommended.

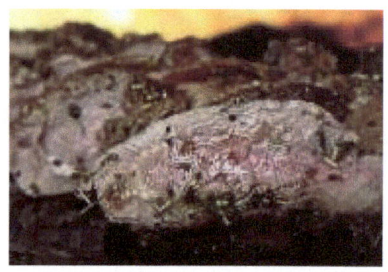

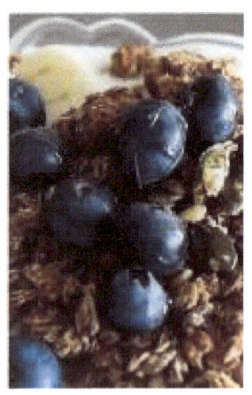

Carbohydrates

Carbohydrates provide energy, but too many will be stored as fat, so have 1/3 of your daily carb intake about 1 to 1 ½ hours before training and the rest after, so you will have energy to perform in training but the carbs will not be stored as fat.

Healthy Fats

Healthy fats include olive oil, flaxseeds, nuts and nut butters, CLA and fish oil acids

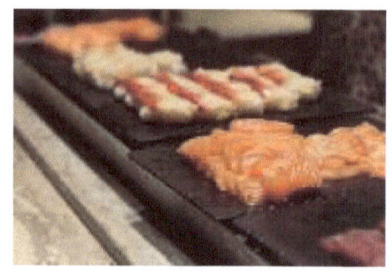

Get about 20 to 30 grams of these daily.

Vegetables

Vegetables can be your greatest assets in increasing caloric intake, satisfying the appetite and losing body fat, even while building muscle

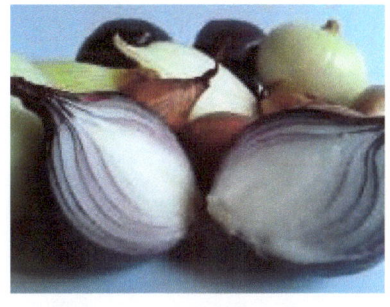

They offer key nutrients and energy. Eat them with each meal and the more the better, think pounds not ounces.

Final Thoughts

Weight lifting to gain strength and muscle requires discipline, patience, motivation, and most of all perseverance, but the end results and benefits are well worth it.

Weight lifting is an integral and important part of a well-balanced approach to health, and fitness that will serve you well into old age.

Any woman who wants to increase lean muscle mass, lower

their percentage of body fat and gain strength would be well advised to add weight training exercises to their normal workout routine.

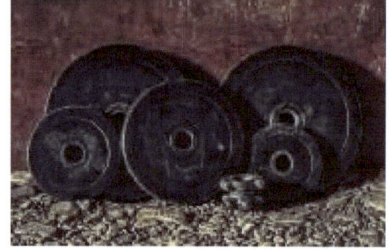

When you train hard and with great intensity and allow for ample rest and recovery time, you will gain the body of your dreams.

Cardio + Strength + Muscle Mass + Nutrition = Sound Fitness

Push hard and you will get phenomenal results, see you at the gym ladies!

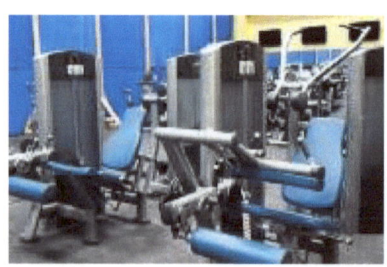

Other Relevant Fitness Books by This Author

If you would like to read more about fitness and strength training, here is a list of the titles, CreateSpace links and descriptions:

https://www.createspace.com/6481324

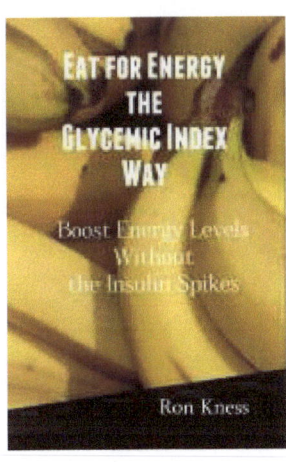

- Are you tired of feeling tired? If you find it hard to concentrate and focus, or you are feeling lifeless and worn out, there is a solution.

In my book we explore how to boost and sustain energy levels from meal to meal by choosing foods using the Glycemic Index scale.

Also, you'll…
• Learn About the Link Between the Amount of Carbs You Eat and How Much Energy You Have During the Day
• Find Out Why Complex Carbs Are Better for Long-Term Energy
• Discover the Disastrous Effect of Sugar on Your Energy
• Determine the Best Types of Breakfasts for Staying Energized All Day Long
• Uncover Foods That Rob You of Your Energy
• Realize How Foods That Are Easier to Digest Give

You More Energy
• Hear How Stimulants Such as Coffee Don't Really Energize You
• Reveal The Best Type of Carbs to Eat as a Pre-Workout Snack
• See Why Filling Up on Fiber Can Be a Great Way to Get More Energy
• Master Feeling Full Without Over Eating
• Become an Expert in Maintaining Good Energy Throughout the Day by Focusing on Your Diet

This book makes it really simple to adjust your diet- no fuss, no complicated ingredients, no unattainable goals. Everyone can use the information from this book and apply it to their own, individual routine and still achieve amazing results!

https://www.createspace.com/6114822

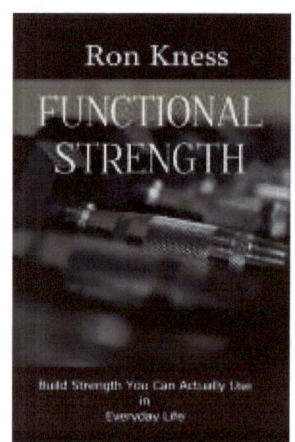

Health and fitness fads come and go all the time but unfortunately not all of them are worth your time and effort. Some of them don't work, some of them are over-hyped and some of them are just plain dangerous.

But 'functional strength' is different. While functional strength is very much in vogue right now, it's not a 'fad' by any means. In fact, functional strength is the opposite of a fad and it's a step in the right direction for all of fitness.

That's because functional strength take it all back: takes it all back to the reasons that most of us started training in the first place. Or at least the reasons we should be training.

When you train for functional strength and fitness, everything becomes easier: from opening a jam jar, to helping a friend move furniture, to getting out of bed in the morning.

And if you want to train for your appearance as your first priority? Well then this is still the right way to go: because when you train for strength and power, you look much better. Don't believe me?

Then think about it logically: the reason that humans find healthy people attractive is because we assume they have better genetics and are better able to protect themselves and their families. Someone with functional strength really can do all those things and really is healthier – so they send all of those unconscious signals that make them more attractive to the opposite sex!

Learn how to build strength that will not only improve everyday life, but also your appearance.

https://www.createspace.com/6622994

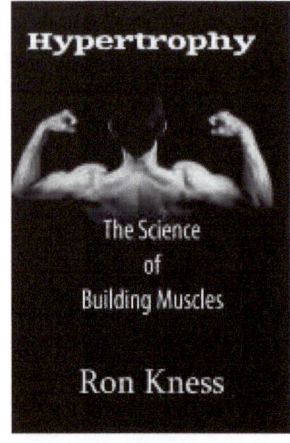

Discover the secrets to muscle growth, supreme strength and maintaining a healthy diet!

So how on Earth are you going to magically build muscle?

Well, actually there is no magic. Unless you count powerful information as magic (and you should), there is no spells and magic potions here.

Instead, we are going to replace magic with a structured plan that if you follow, will lead to incredible results.

What you'll discover in this Book:

- The difference between fast and slow twitch muscle fiber

- The difference between 'sarcoplasmic' and 'myofibrillar' hypertrophy

- How to combine different types of training to experience 'athletic aesthetics'

- Why both compound AND isolation movements are perfectly valid

- How to train faster for better results

- How to use the Joe Weider intensity principles

- How to see growth even as a 'hard gainer'

- How to become incredibly lean and ripped, even as an endomorph - a person who has a hard time gaining weight

- How to work out your 'training philosophy'

- How to choose a fitness movement that works for you

- ...and much, much more!

This book will tell you everything you need to know to get into the gym tomorrow and start building a new body.

https://www.createspace.com/6295221

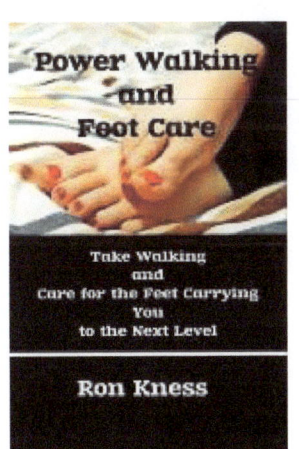

With Power Walking, you perform exaggerated walking movements. It doesn't have a very high impact on your feet. Secondly, you do it very fast without running. So, it's like running except you don't pound your joints like you do with running.

It's a fun, doctor-recommended form of exercise that almost anyone can do no matter their physical condition at the time.

The second part of the book is taking care of your feet. It addresses common foot conditions along with foot issues from diabetes and Plantar Fasciitis.

Learn how to take care of your feet so that you can join those who are converting over to power walking.

About the Author

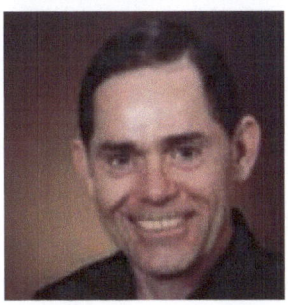

I grew up in Central Minnesota, where my parents owned and operated a fishing resort. Once out of high school I tried a couple of semesters of college, only to quit halfway through the Spring term; I decided at that time that college wasn't for me.

Then I decided to follow my father's previous occupation as an auto mechanic. I graduated from a two-year of vocational training course and worked as a mechanic for five years. While in vocational training, I decided to join the National Guard where I eventually ended up working full-time for 32 years.

So how does all of this relate to writing? In one of my leadership schools, the instructor, who was an English teacher at a juvenile detention center, presented writing to me in a whole new way - a way that started to develop my interest in working with words.

I eventually went back to college on the GI Bill while I was working and earned my Bachelor's degree in Business Administration. Taking a class or two per semester at night and on weekends took me seven years to complete my degree.

Fast forward about 40 years and I now have published over 75 books on Amazon for Kindle, CreateSpace and other publishing platforms.

Besides my own writing, I also ghostwrite ebooks, reports, articles, blogs and do Kindle conversions for clients on a variety of topics.

Today my wife and I are retired from our careers and live in Gold Canyon, AZ. I now write as a retirement business where you'll find me happily sitting in my office typing away on my laptop as I work on my next book or ghostwriting project . . . that is if we are not traveling on a cruise ship - our new-found mode of travel.